Tobacco Free Initiative

Regional Action Plan
2005 - 2009

**WORLD HEALTH ORGANIZATION
WESTERN PACIFIC REGION**

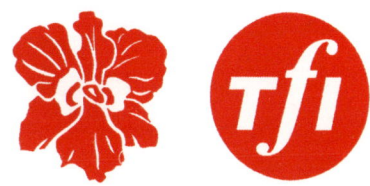

WHO Library Cataloguing in Publication Data

Tobacco free initiative : regional action plan, 2005-2009.

1. Tobacco. 2. Smoking. 3. Tobacco use cessation.

ISBN 92 9061 184 7   (NLM Classification: WM 290)

© World Health Organization 2005

All rights reserved.

The designations employed and the presentation of the material in this publication do not imply the expression of any opinion whatsoever on the part of the World Health Organization concerning the legal status of any country, territory, city or area or of its authorities, or concerning the delimitation of its frontiers or boundaries. Dotted lines on maps represent approximate border lines for which there may not yet be full agreement.

The mention of specific companies or of certain manufacturers' products does not imply that they are endorsed or recommended by the World Health Organization in preference to others of a similar nature that are not mentioned. Errors and omissions excepted, the names of proprietary products are distinguished by initial capital letters.

The World Health Organization does not warrant that the information contained in this publication is complete and correct and shall not be liable for any damages incurred as a result of its use.

Publications of the World Health Organization can be obtained from Marketing and Dissemination, World Health Organization, 20 Avenue Appia, 1211 Geneva 27, Switzerland (tel: +41 22 791 2476; fax: +41 22 791 4857; email: bookorders@who.int). Requests for permission to reproduce WHO publications, in part or in whole, or to translate them – whether for sale or for noncommercial distribution – should be addressed to Publications, at the above address (fax: +41 22 791 4806; email: permissions@who.int). For WHO Western Pacific Regional Publications, request for permission to reproduce should be addressed to Publications Office, World Health Organization, Regional Office for the Western Pacific, P.O. Box 2932, 1000, Manila, Philippines, Fax. No. (632) 521-1036, email: publications@wpro.who.int

Contents

Page

ACKNOWLEDGEMENTS _____ 5

1. INTRODUCTION _____ 9

    1.1 ISSUES _____ 11

    1.2 RESPONSE _____ 17

    1.3 GOAL _____ 20

    1.3 OBJECTIVES _____ 21

2. REGIONAL ACTION PLAN 2005-2009 _____ 21

3. KEY REFERENCES _____ 27

4. KEY RESOURCES _____ 30

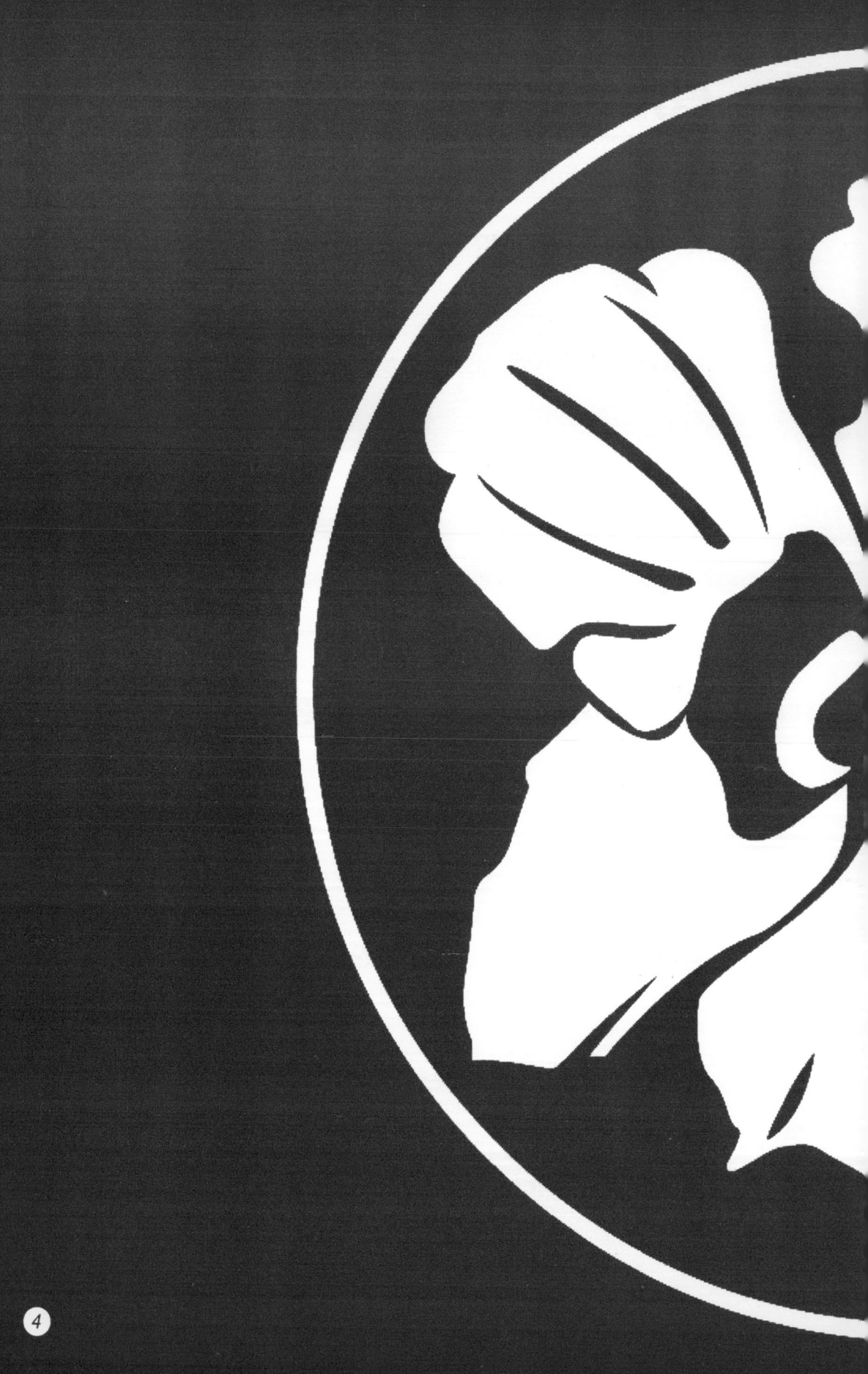

Acknowledgements

The *Tobacco Free Initiative Regional Action Plan (2005-2009)* is the result of year-long intensive development, discussion and consultation with Western Pacific Region Member States, experts and many others.

The initial conceptualization of the Plan is owed to a collaboration between Tobacco Free Initiative (TFI) and Dr Annette M. David. Review of the draft objectives and strategies, and development of specific activities was done at the Third Meeting of National Focal Persons for the Tobacco Free Initiative in Manila, March 2004. In that regard, we recognize the outstanding contributions of the following participants:

National Focal Persons for the Tobacco Free Initiative

Dr Haji Rozaimee Tengah
Ministry of Health
BRUNEI DARUSSALAM

Dr Lim Thai Pheang
National Center for
Health Promotion
CAMBODIA

Dr Li Xinhua
Ministry of Health
CHINA

Dr Henry Kong Wing-ming
Department of Health
HONG KONG (CHINA)

Dr Chan Tan Mui
Center for Disease Control
and Prevention
Health Services
MACAO (CHINA)

Ms Natalie Ngapoko Short
Ministry of Health
COOK ISLANDS

Mr Midion Iohp
Department of Health, Education
and Social Affairs
FEDERATED STATES OF MICRONESIA

Ms Luseane Rai Viliame
Ministry of Health
FIJI

Mr Eugene S.N. Santos
Department of Public Health
and Social Services
GUAM

Dr Tetsuo Hirako
Ministry of Health, Labour and Welfare
JAPAN

Dr Somsy Pasithiphone
Ministry of Health
LAO PEOPLE'S DEMOCRATIC REPUBLIC

Dr Zarihah Moh'd Zain
Ministry of Health
MALAYSIA

Ms Justina R. Langidrik
Ministry of Health
MARSHALL ISLANDS

Dr Gombodoryiin Tsetsegdary
Ministry of Health
MONGOLIA

Acknowledgements

Dr Jean-Paul Grangeon
Chef du Service des Actions Sanitaires
NEW CALEDONIA

Mr Graeme Gillespie
Ministry of Health
NEW ZEALAND

Dr Sylvia Andres
Ministry of Health
PALAU

Dr James Wangi
Department of Health
PAPUA NEW GUINEA

Dr Ma. Alicia Jessica de Leon
Department of Health
PHILIPPINES

Dr Yoon-Jeong Shin
Korea Institute for Health and
Social Affairs
REPUBLIC OF KOREA

Mr Ilyong Son
Ministry of Health & Welfare
REPUBLIC OF KOREA

Dr Herbert Peters
Tupua Tamasese Meaole Hospital
SAMOA

Ms Choo Lin
Health Promotion Board
SINGAPORE

Dr George Wilson Malefoasi
Ministry of Health
SOLOMON ISLANDS

Mr Jean-Jacques Rory
Ministry of Health
VANUATU

Dr Nguyen Trong Khoa
Ministry of Health
VIET NAM

*CONSULTANTS, TEMPORARY ADVISERS
REPRESENTATIVES / OBSERVERS*

Mr Stephen Tamplin

Mr Matthew Allen
Allen and Clarke Policy and
Regulatory Specialists
New Zealand

Ms Belinda Hughes
PATH Canada

Dr Caleb Otto

Young Ja Lee, RN, Ph.D
Korean Association of Smoking and
Health

Ms Estela Montejo
Department of Finance, Philippines

Ms Luz Tagunicar
Department of Health, Philippines

Dr Marina Baquilod
National Epidemiology Center
Philippines

Acknowledgements

Dr Florante Trinidad
Department of Health, Philippines

Dr Carmelita C. Canila
Framework Convention Alliance, Philippines

Ms Josefina de la Cuadra
Philippine Health Insurance

Ms Marita V. Pasuengos
City State Centre Philippines

Dr Harley Stanton
The Secretariat of the Pacific Community

Dr Sohei Makino
Tokyo Allergic Research Institute

Dr Kewu Huang
WHO Collaborating Centre for Tobacco or Health

SECRETARIAT

Mr Burke Fishburn
WHO Western Pacific Regional Office

Mr Jonathan Santos
WHO Western Pacific Regional Office

Mr Gregory Hallen
WHO Cambodia

Dr Yanwei Wu
WHO China

Ms Nancy MacDonald
WHO Samoa

Dr Max De Courten
WHO South Pacific

Dr Nguyen Tuan Lam
WHO Viet Nam

Dr Susan Mercado
WHO Western Pacific Regional Office

Dr Gauden Galea
WHO Western Pacific Regional Office

Dr Graham Harrison
WHO Western Pacific Regional Office

Dr Frank Mueke
WHO Western Pacific Regional Office

Dr Pieter Van Maaren
WHO Western Pacific Regional Office

Mr Dorjsuren Bayarsaikhan
WHO Western Pacific Regional Office

Ms Anjana Bhushan
WHO Western Pacific Regional Office

Dr Vera da Costa e Silva
WHO Headquarters, Geneva

In finalizing the document, we are also grateful for the expert review of Dr Judith Mackay, Asia Consultancy on Tobacco Control, and Mrs Anne S. Blackwood, United States Department of State. Finally, we wish to acknowledge the outstanding commitment and support of the ministers of health, who endorsed this plan at the fifty-fifth session of the WHO Regional Committee for the Wesrtern Pacific in Shanghai, China, 13-17 September 2004.

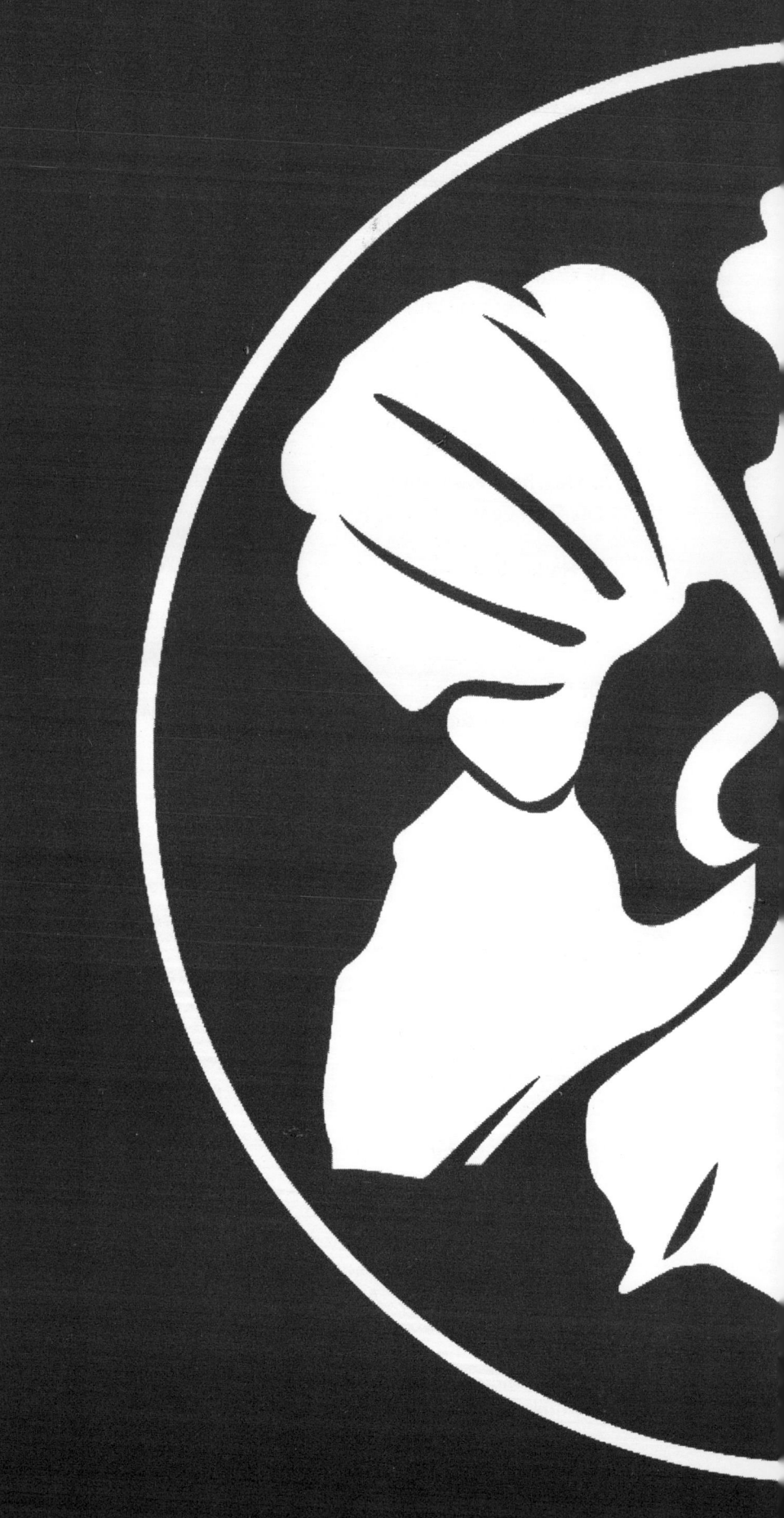

Introduction

The Regional Action Plan for the Tobacco Free Initiative (TFI) 2005-2009 contains the vision and strategic plan for tobacco control in the Western Pacific Region for the next five years. The previous action plans, covering the periods 1990-1994, 1995-1999, and 2000-2004, provide the foundation for this plan.

Based on the recommendations of the Third Meeting of National Focal Persons for the Tobacco Free Initiative (2004), this document builds on the previous plans and highlights the importance of increasing and sustaining momentum for effective tobacco control by:

1. attaining the timely ratification of the WHO Framework Convention on Tobacco Control (WHO FCTC or "the Convention") among Western Pacific Region Member States through a coordinated regional strategy, thus contributing towards the Convention's entry into force; and,

2. further enhancing the capacity of Member States to successfully implement the provisions of the Convention and effectively address the tobacco epidemic.

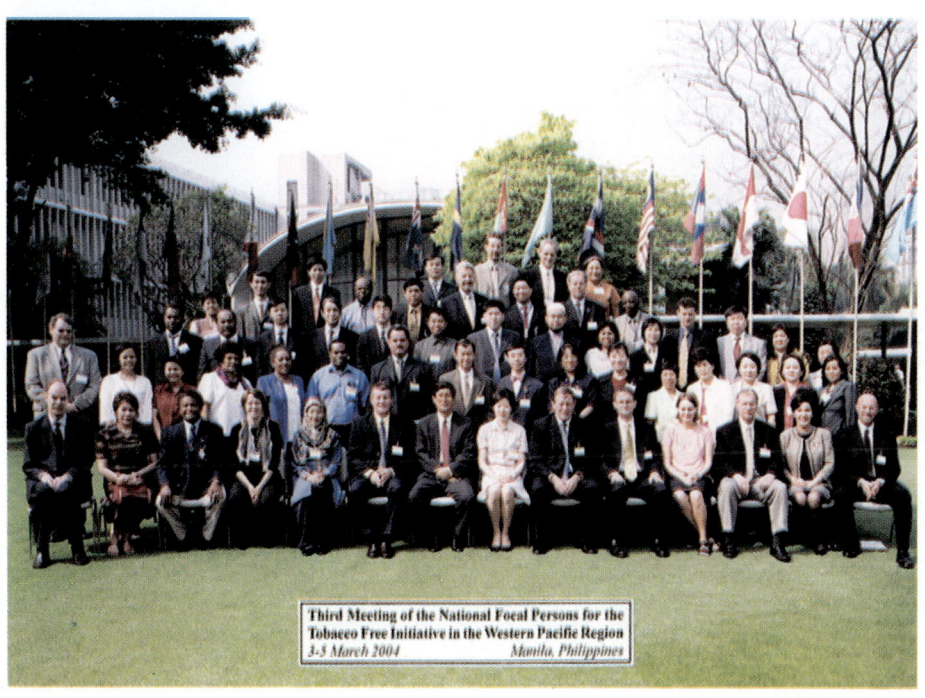

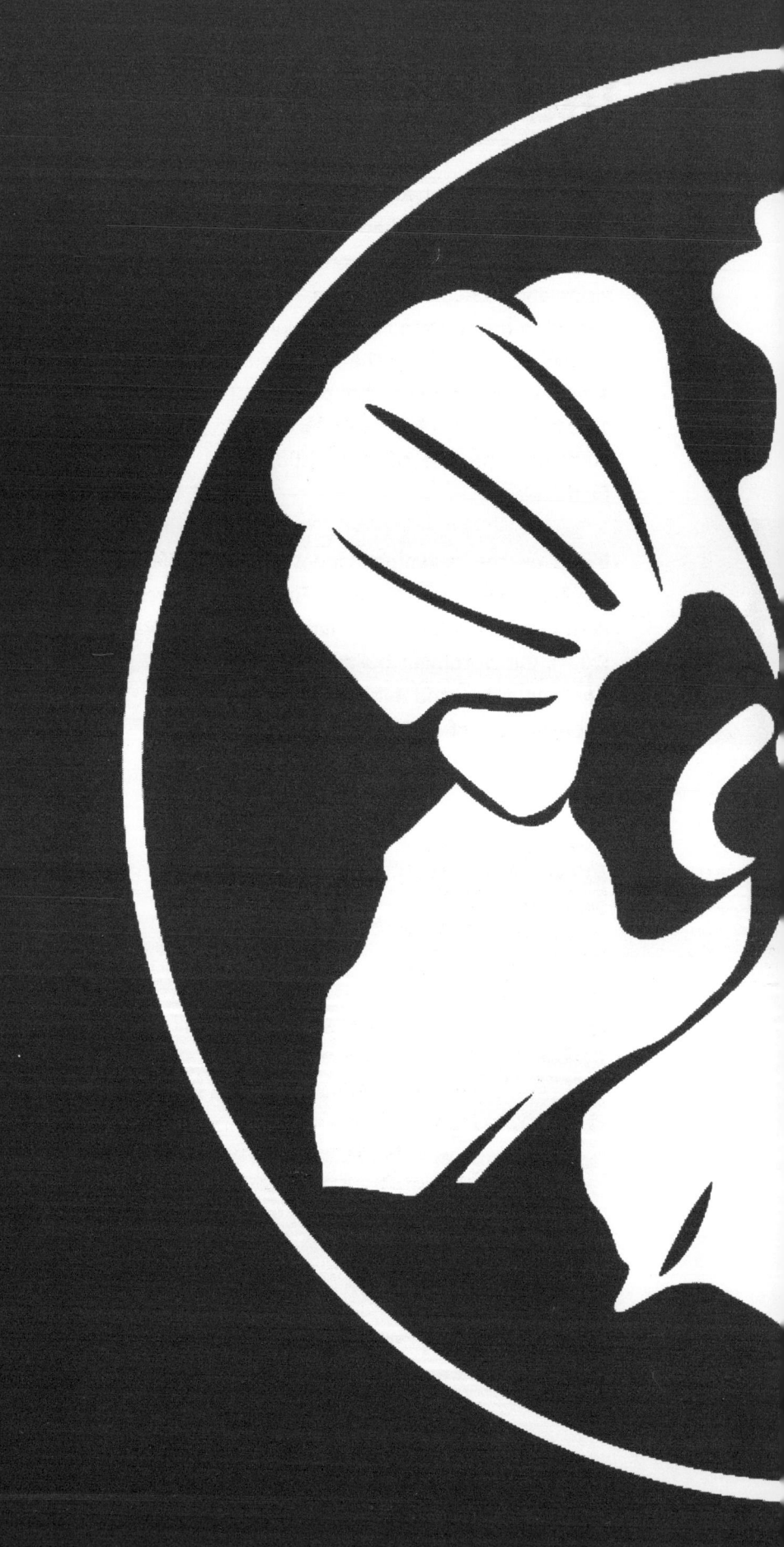

Issues

The tobacco epidemic is likely the greatest tragedy in public health. Already, tobacco kills one in ten persons globally, accounting for approximately 5 million deaths per year. Western Pacific Region Member States bear a disproportionate burden of tobacco-related mortality, as the Region accounts for 20% of these deaths.

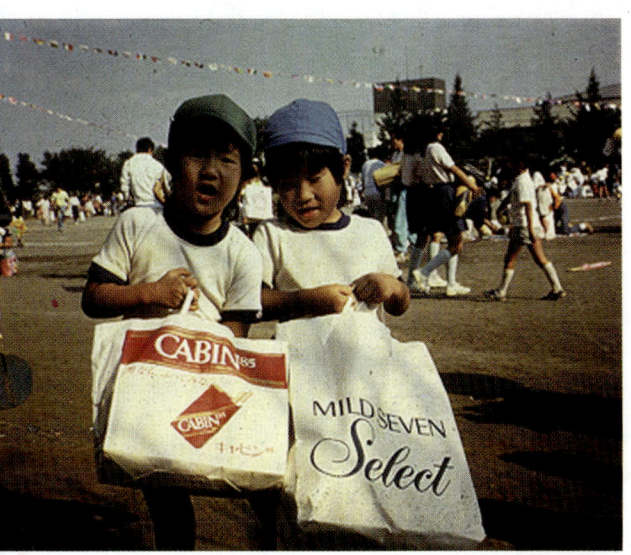

Tobacco use is also a major contributor to the Region's disease burden. In both developed and developing countries within the Region, tobacco consumption causes or aggravates several chronic diseases that together comprise up to 18% of the total disability adjusted life-years (DALYs) lost. These estimates do not include the years of healthy life lost by non-smokers whose health is compromised by exposure to second-hand smoke. Moreover, the long lead time between exposure to tobacco smoke and the development of clinical disease, and the rapidly increasing pool of young smokers in the Western Pacific imply that the consequences of tobacco use within the Region will be far greater in the future, unless action is taken immediately to curb tobacco use.

Much of the disease burden and premature mortality that are attributable to tobacco use disproportionately affect the poor. Worldwide, poor and uneducated men are more likely to smoke than men with higher incomes or education. In those countries where reliable data on mortality exist, much of the excess mortality of poor and less-educated men can be attributed to smoking. Furthermore, smokers who live in low and middle-income countries quit less often.

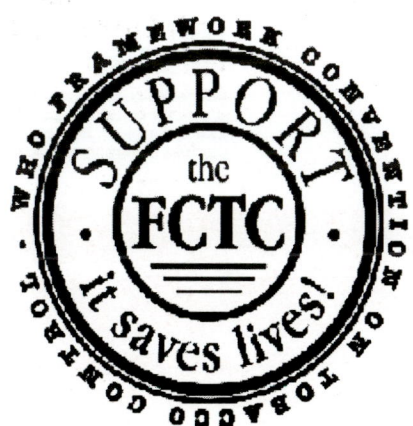

Issues

Poverty and tobacco use are linked in other ways. Several studies have shown that in the poorest households of some low-income countries, as much as 10%-17% of total household expenditure is on tobacco. This means that impoverished families have less money to spend on essential items such as food, health care and education. Indeed, tobacco's role in exacerbating poverty has not been fully elucidated, and requires greater scrutiny.

The economic costs to society of tobacco use are staggering. The high price of treating tobacco-related diseases is compounded by productivity losses. Smokers are less productive workers, due to increased sickness. Deaths from tobacco often occur during the productive years of life, depleting a nation's workforce.

In addition, concern among Western Pacific Region Member States is escalating regarding the increasing numbers of women and children exposed to the harm of tobacco. Already, a number of Pacific island countries have extremely high rates of tobacco use, involving both chewing and smoking, among their women. Recent data from the Global Youth Tobacco Survey (GYTS) indicate a disturbing high rate of tobacco use, and early age of initiation, among the Region's youth. A separate issue involves the countless numbers of women and children who are exposed to second-hand smoke, particularly in countries such as Cambodia, China, the Philippines and Viet Nam, where smoking rates among men are extremely high.

The addictive properties of nicotine make cessation difficult, even for those tobacco users who are highly motivated to quit. This, coupled with the lack of effective cessation guidelines and programmes in many Western Pacific Region countries, particularly addressing the issue of chewing tobacco, and the high cost of pharmacologic treatment for nicotine addiction, are challenges that Member States need to address.

Response

All these factors make tobacco control an urgent public health priority, especially among the developing countries of the Western Pacific. Western Pacific Region Member States recognize the gravity of the Region's tobacco epidemic, and affirm the need for effective and immediate action to curb tobacco consumption.

Evidence-based measures to reduce tobacco consumption exist, and are proving effective in several Western Pacific Region Member States that have developed and implemented strong national tobacco control programmes, such as Australia, New Zealand and Singapore. Several other countries in the Region that have begun country-level tobacco control are discovering that weak or inconsistent enforcement of tobacco control policies and laws renders these measures ineffective. The situation is compounded by the globalization of tobacco trade, advertising and marketing, which very often are beyond the reach of even the strongest national policies and laws.

The globalization of the tobacco epidemic necessitates a coordinated response by countries. WHO's Member States successfully negotiated the final text of the WHO Framework Convention on Tobacco Control at the sixth session of the Intergovernmental Negotiating Body in Geneva, Switzerland, in February 2003 and the Fifty-sixth World Health Assembly adopted the text in May 2003. As of 1 December 2004, the required 40 Member States had ratified the Convention enabling it to enter into force on 27 February 2005. The Convention will now be able to help countries to reduce tobacco use and the years of healthy life lost due to tobacco.

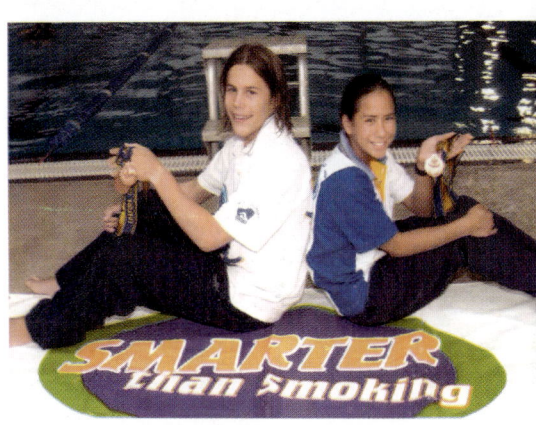

While the Convention provides guidelines to reduce the harm from tobacco, definitive action to control tobacco must take place at the national level. Therefore, the success of the Convention will depend almost entirely on the ability of countries to implement and enforce its provisions. Further enhancing national capacity must take place at the same time as efforts to ensure that the Convention is ratified, because Member States need to be ready for implementation when it enters into force. This requires long-term political commitment to developing and sustaining country capacity, and to identifying and appropriating the resources needed for comprehensive tobacco control.

Response

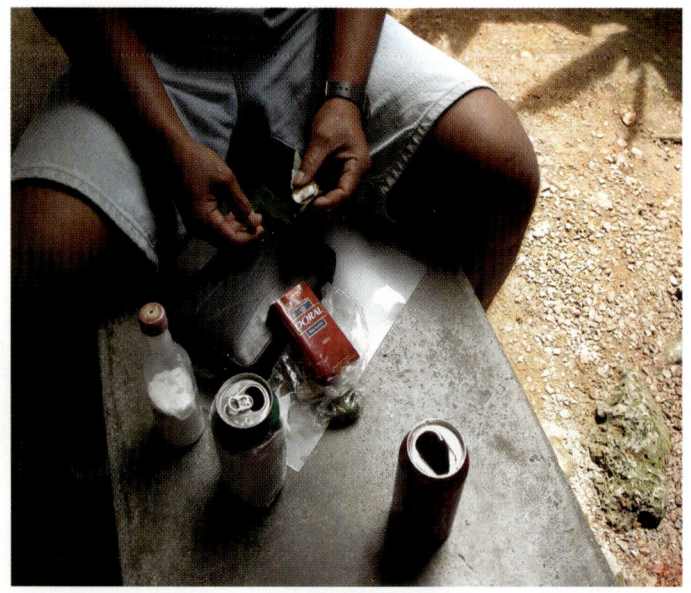

Ensuring the sustainability of tobacco control programmes remains a major challenge for many countries, and must be given priority. The tobacco industry provides much of the opposition. Attempts by the tobacco industry to oppose or circumvent national and regional tobacco control efforts may escalate as the entry into force of the Convention nears. Therefore, to safeguard the Convention and strengthen national tobacco control efforts strategic collaboration is needed with other health programmes, development and poverty alleviation initiatives, as well as with diverse sectors within governments, related international agencies and nongovernmental organizations (NGOs).

Exploring means to finance national activities intended to achieve the objective of the Convention should be actively pursued, such as through tobacco taxes, the creation of a special fund, or other appropriate mechanisms, in accordance with national plans, priorities and programmes. In addition, all relevant potential and existing resources, financial, technical, or otherwise, both public and private that are available for tobacco control activities, should be mobilized and utilized for the benefit of all Parties to the Convention, especially developing countries and countries with economies in transition.

Member States need to coordinate their efforts to address those aspects of the tobacco epidemic that transcend national borders. A major issue involves trade liberalization as it applies to tobacco products. Other transnational issues include cross-country illicit trade in tobacco products, global marketing and advertising. Developing subregional and regional mechanisms to effectively deal with these transnational issues is addressed by this plan of action.

Response

Tracking efforts to curb the tobacco epidemic must be done systematically at both the national and regional levels. Standard surveillance instruments and methods are needed to enable Member States to monitor progress in achieving real and measurable health impacts. Finally, a regional strategy to guide research and the generation of evidence to support policy and programme development is necessary throughout the entire process of tobacco control capacity building. This should be accompanied by a coordinated mechanism for evaluation, advocacy and information dissemination to the relevant audiences, enabling all Member States to gain access to critical data and facilitating information exchange within the Region.

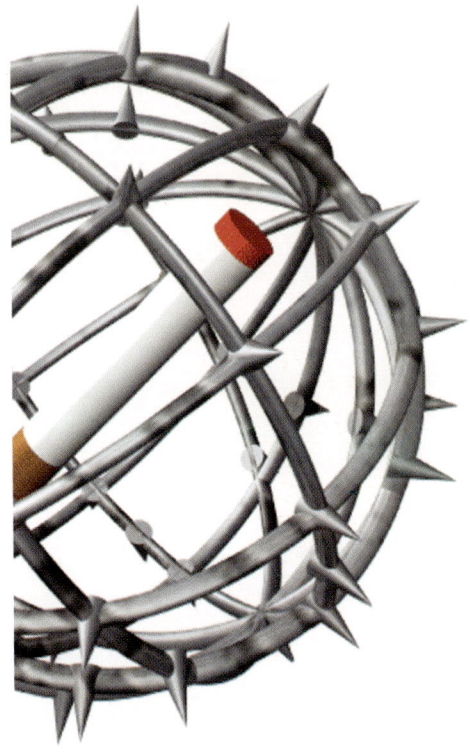

Goal

The goal of this action plan is to significantly reduce the burden of disease and death caused by tobacco, through a substantial reduction in the prevalence of tobacco use, exposure to tobacco smoke and disparities related to tobacco use and its effects.

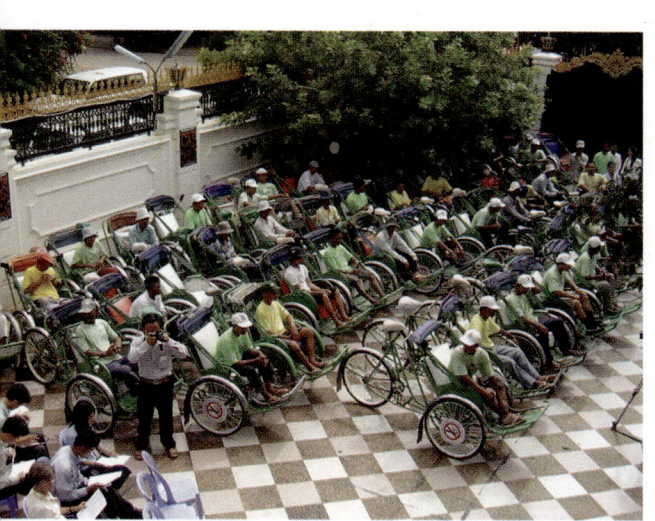

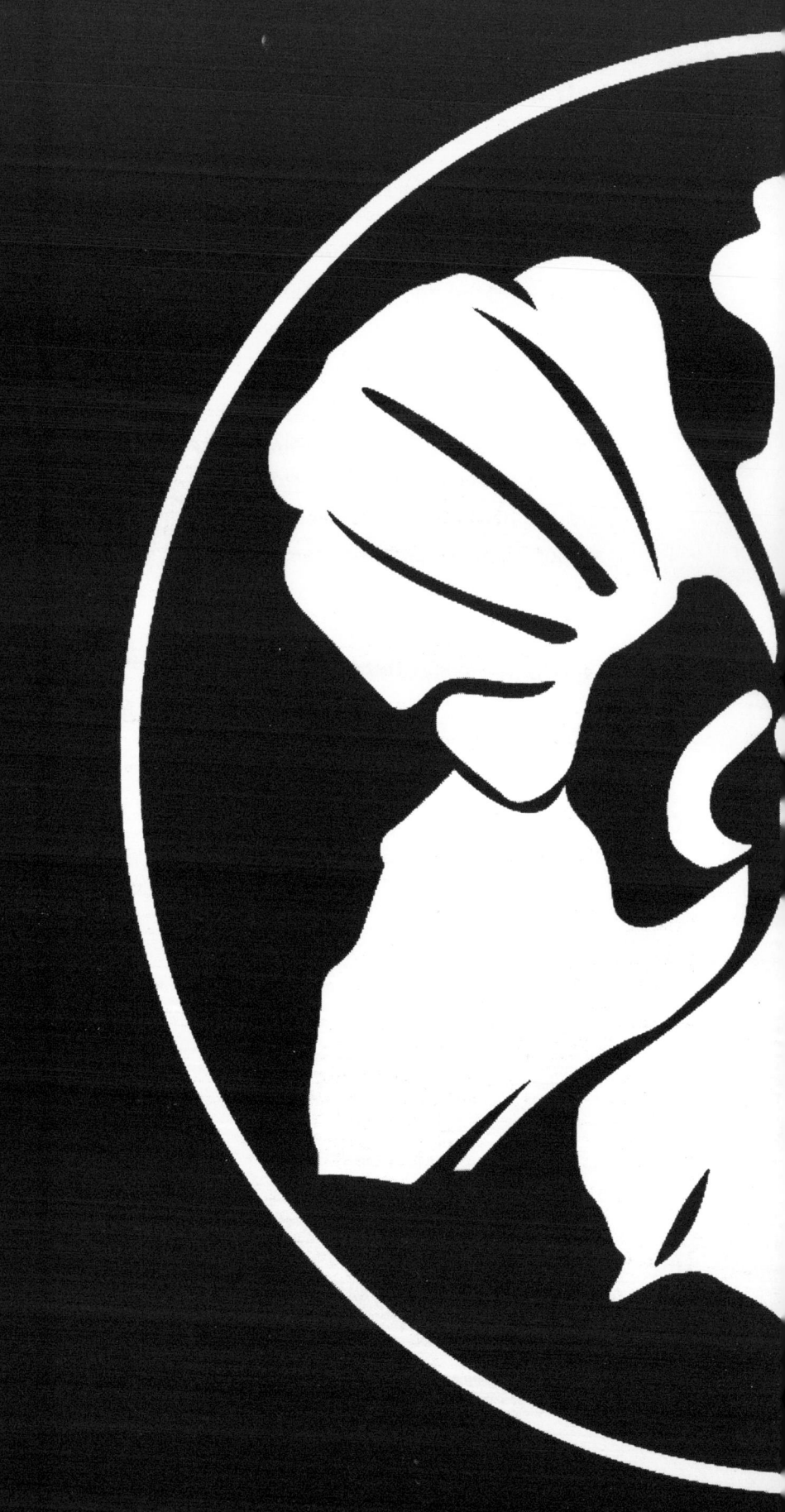

Objectives

By 2009:

1. Attain ratification of the WHO Framework Convention on Tobacco Control (WHO FCTC or "the Convention") in all Western Pacific Region (WPR) Member States

2. Strengthen national capacity for tobacco control to enable implementation of comprehensive tobacco control strategies in an effective and sustainable manner in at least 80% (29) of WPR Member States and areas

3. Develop and formally adopt measures to ensure sustainability of tobacco control programmes in all WPR Member States and areas

4. Establish Regional, subregional and national mechanisms to address transnational tobacco control issues

5. Enhance surveillance, research, information dissemination and advocacy across the Region

The following table provides the details of the Tobacco Free Initiative's Regional Action Plan 2005-2009, including examples of strategic actions that may be taken.

OBJECTIVE 1:	By 2009, attain ratification of the WHO FCTC in all WPR Member States
Expected Result 1.1	***Entry into force of the WHO FCTC***
Indicator 1.1.1	***Number of WPR Member States that ratify the Convention***
Strategic actions for Member States	***Strategic actions for WHO***
Increase awareness of the specific obligations contained in the WHO FCTC, its opportunities and implications, and the process of ratification and implementation among key decision-makers and bodies that will be involved in the decision and process to ratify the Convention	Continue to provide technical assistance to Member States on the WHO FCTC, its opportunities and implications to countries, and the process of ratification and implementation
Collaborate with partners in the public and private sector to create and implement an advocacy campaign for the ratification of the WHO FCTC	Inform WPR Member States about and facilitate their participation in regional and global advocacy campaigns for the WHO FCTC ratification

Objective 2

OBJECTIVE 2:	By 2009, strengthen national capacity for tobacco control to enable implementation of comprehensive tobacco control strategies in an effective and sustainable manner in at least 80% (29) of WPR Member States and areas
Expected result 2.1	WPR Member States with established national tobacco control programmes increased from 2004 baseline
Indicators:	
2.1.1	Number of Member States with staff dedicated to tobacco control
2.1.2	Number of Member States with officially designated national tobacco control programmes
Expected result 2.2	WPR Member States with comprehensive tobacco control policies and national plans of action increased from 2004 baseline
Indicators:	
2.2.1	Number of WPR Member States with national plans of action consistent with Articles 6 to 14 of the WHO FCTC
2.2.2	Number of WPR Member States with national policies and legislation that reflect the key strategies outlined in the WHO FCTC
2.2.3	Number of WPR Member States with clearly articulated strategies to target high-risk and potentially hard-to-reach populations

Strategic actions for Member States	*Strategic actions for WHO*
Establish national tobacco control programmes with dedicated staff, if none exists, or strengthen existing national tobacco control programmes	Identify Member States with no existing national tobacco control programmes and provide technical assistance for the establishment of these programmes
Review existing national plans of action and tobacco control policies and legislation, and amend these, as appropriate, to reflect the WHO FCTC provisions, as a minimum standard for a comprehensive approach to tobacco control. If no action plans, policies or legislation exist, develop new ones that are consistent with or are more stringent than the WHO FCTC	Support technical training and assistance to selected countries (particularly those with demonstrated need and political and programmatic readiness/commitment) for capacity building in tobacco control infrastructure and policy development, and comprehensive approaches consistent with the WHO FCTC
Identify and advocate for evidence-based practices suitable for local conditions	Review and collect best practice models and templates that are applicable to WPR Member States (e.g. cessation strategies applicable to the Region), and develop mechanisms for disseminating these in an efficient and timely manner
Integrate tobacco control approaches into health and education curricula. For example, ensure that appropriate cessation strategies are included in training programmes for health care service providers at all levels	Assist Member States to adapt international guidelines for integrating tobacco control into the health curricula for local use
Formulate targeted strategies to cover high-risk and hard-to-reach populations, especially the poor and underserved, whose tobacco use rates are significant	Disseminate global strategies and best-practice examples that address gender issues, high-risk and hard-to-reach populations and poverty as they relate to tobacco control

Objective 3

OBJECTIVE 3:	**Develop and formally adopt measures to ensure sustainability of tobacco control programmes in all WPR Member States and areas**
Expected Result 3.1	**Tobacco control approaches integrated into public health and other programmes and events**

Indicators:

3.1.1 Number of Member States with multisectoral national committees that coordinate the integration of tobacco control approaches into other health and non-health programmes

3.1.2 Number of Member States that integrate tobacco use prevention and cessation into health promotion, risk reduction and disease control programmes

3.1.3 Number of Member States that incorporate tobacco control policies and interventions into other related non-health programmes, such as development or poverty alleviation

3.1.4 Number of Regional events that incorporate tobacco control policies and approaches

Expected Result 3.2	**Strategies to ensure sustainability of tobacco control programmes operational in Member States**

Indicators:

3.2.1 Number of WPR Member States with national budgets for tobacco control

3.2.2 Number of WPR Member States with mechanisms to channel resources and funding to tobacco control programmes

3.2.3 Extent of international resources committed to supporting tobacco control among WPR Member States

Strategic actions for Member States	*Strategic actions for WHO*
Establish, if none exists, a multisectoral committee to address tobacco control issues at the national level, as well as cross-border issues; if such a body already exists, review and strengthen the composition of the committee	Disseminate guidelines for establishing and sustaining national multisectoral tobacco control committees
Identify and utilize existing opportunities to merge tobacco control policies and interventions into related health and non-health programmes, such as those that address poverty alleviation and sustainable development. For example, Pacific island countries may explore how to incorporate tobacco control into the Healthy Islands initiative	Develop guidelines for integrating tobacco control into other WHO health programmes, such as Non-Communicable Diseases (NCD), Healthy Settings, Tuberculosis and Health Promotion programmes, as well as for other relevant non-health programmes such as those that address development and poverty alleviation
Develop national guidelines for ensuring smoke-free environments in various settings and national and local events	Coordinate and expedite efforts by Member States to incorporate tobacco control policies into national events, and regional and global events held in the Western Pacific, such as the South East Asian Games and the 2008 Olympics in Beijing, China

Objective 3 Continuation

(Obj. 3 con't)	*Develop and formally adopt measures to ensure sustainability of tobacco control programmes in all WPR Member States and areas*
Strategic actions for Member States	*Strategic actions for WHO*
Develop administrative and legislative measures to augment funding and support to the national tobacco control programme, consistent with Article 26, which requires that each Party shall provide financial support for national tobacco control activities, and that the Parties agree that all relevant potential and existing resources should be mobilized and utilized	Identify, collate, systematically review and disseminate models for ensuring sustainability of tobacco control national programmes, with particular emphasis on those that currently exist in some WPR Member States and areas such as Australia, Guam, and New Zealand
Consistent with Article 26, advocate for tobacco control funding from national budget appropriations/allocations	Provide technical assistance and support to countries who want to legislate measures that will ensure sustained funding for tobacco control
Advocate to bilateral and multilateral donors to allocate funds and resources for tobacco control, whether directly or as a component of funding grants to related programmes such as health services development, health promotion, tuberculosis, sustainable development, healthy environments	Coordinate external support for tobacco control from international agencies and other partners for WPR Member States
Strengthen social mobilization and community participation in tobacco control activities through, for example, information and education campaigns and implementation of national smokefree policies	Provide technical assistance and other support to countries to promote social mobilization and community participation in tobacco control activities

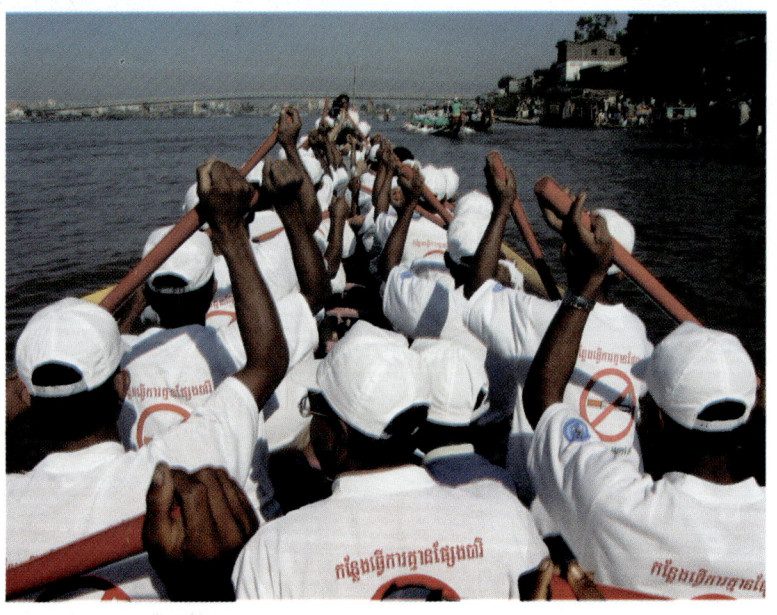

Objective 4

OBJECTIVE 4:	Establish Regional, subregional and national mechanisms to address transnational tobacco control issues
Expected result 4.1	**Bilateral/multilateral partnerships established to address transnational tobacco control issues**

Indicators:
4.1.1   Number of national, subregional and regional networks/alliances working on transnational tobacco control issues
4.1.2   Number of subregional and regional meetings that include transnational tobacco control issues on their agenda

Expected result 4.2	**Multisectoral strategies in support of tobacco control developed**

Indicators:
4.2.1   Number of interventions focusing on trade, economic, legislative, environmental, developmental and regulatory mechanisms to deal with transnational issues in actual use within the Region

Strategic actions for Member States	Strategic actions for WHO
Identify potential partners nationally, within, and outside the Region that share common concerns regarding transnational tobacco control issues	Assist Member States to establish alliances and networks that will enable them to respond more effectively to cross-border tobacco control issues at the regional and international level
Advocate for the inclusion of tobacco control transnational issues on the agenda of national, subregional and Regional bodies, such as national multisectoral coordinating committees for tobacco control, ASEAN, the Pacific Forum, Pacific Island Health Officers Association (PIHOA), and Secretariat for the Pacific Community (SPC)	Support subregional tobacco control activities among Member States with common interests and concerns
Develop and enforce collaborative interventions with neighbouring countries to regulate tobacco products and reduce the cross-border illegal trade, promotion and advertising of tobacco products	Convene a biregional meeting with WHO's South-East Asia Regional Office (SEARO) to tackle cross-border issues, particularly smuggling and harmonizing tobacco product regulation

Objective 5

OBJECTIVE 5	**Enhance surveillance, research, evaluation, information dissemination and advocacy across the Region, and globally**
Expected Result 5.1	**A set of standard global/Regional surveillance and evaluation instruments and methodologies utilized by all WPR Member States and areas**
Indicator:	
5.1.1	Number of Member States that complete standardized global/regional tobacco control surveys such as the Global Youth Tobacco Survey (GYTS)
Expected result 5.2	**Regional and national tobacco control research agendas developed and under implementation**
Indicator:	
5.2.1	Number of WPR Member States implementing research projects that address local needs, such as the link between tobacco use and poverty, and interventions to reduce chewing tobacco
Expected result 5.3	**A mechanism for disseminating information available to all WPR Member States and areas**
Indicators:	
5.3.1	Number of WPR Member States and areas covered by the Global Information System on Tobacco Control (GISTC)
5.3.2	Number of average monthly "hits" for the Tobacco Free Initiative website
Expected Result 5.4	**Increased public awareness of the tobacco epidemic and tobacco industry activities**
Indicators:	
5.4.1	Number of WPR Member States that have local organizations in both the public and private sectors undertaking media/educational campaigns on the harmful effects of tobacco use
5.4.2	Number of WPR Member States that participate in annual World No Tobacco Day (WNTD) activities and other events highlighting the need for action against the tobacco epidemic
5.4.3	Number of WPR Member States that monitor tobacco industry activities

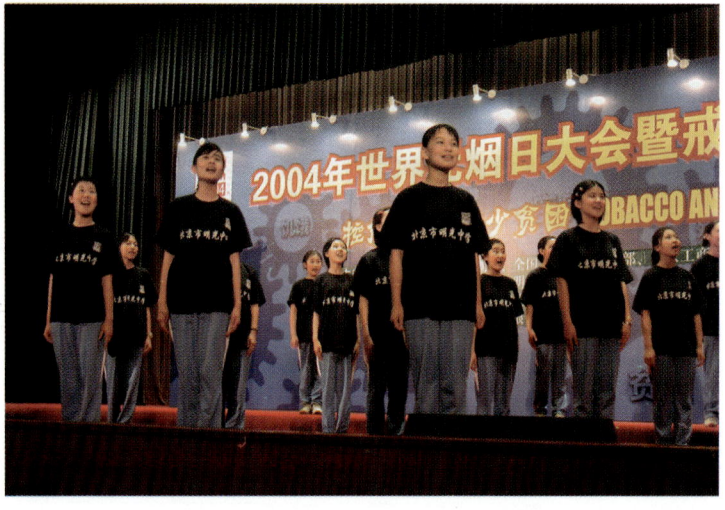

Objective 5 Continuation

(Obj. 5 con't)	**Enhance surveillance, research, evaluation, information dissemination and advocacy across the Region, and globally**
Strategic actions for Member States	*Strategic actions for WHO*
Regularly implement standard global/regional surveys and evaluation on tobacco control activities and promptly report results to the WHO Regional office	Develop and disseminate standard global/regional surveillance and evaluation instruments and methods, train Member States to utilize these, and collect all data from Member States
Develop and implement a research agenda that addresses local needs and data gaps, including: (a) initiating an analysis of the relationship between tobacco use and poverty; and, (b) evaluating interventions to help reduce chewing tobacco use	Assist Member States to develop relevant and practical research agendas to support tobacco control and to submit the results of research projects for peer review and publication
Create a national database for tobacco control that includes information taken from other existing sources of data, such as school surveys and national household surveys	Coordinate data collection from other related health surveys, such as STEPwise approach to surveillance (STEPS) and the Behaviour Risk Factor Survey (BRFS)
Regularly report to the Regional Office, so that country profiles are updated on the Regional online database	Improve the WPR online database, and work with HQ and other Regional Offices to develop a standard global online database
Develop and implement a mechanism to disseminate pertinent information to local policy-makers, stakeholders and other key partners, including development agencies	Expand the existing Regional Research Clearinghouse (currently based at Universiti Sains Malay, Penang, Malaysia) and fully utilize the Regional TFI website to ensure timely dissemination of information to all WPR Member States and areas, and partners
Communicate and share information with other Member States who have similar concerns	Promote active information exchange among partners and Member States
Encourage local organizations in both the public and private sectors to undertake evidence-based media/educational campaigns on the harmful effects of tobacco use	Facilitate collaboration between non governmental organizations and other civil society bodies with TFI programmes at the national, subregional and Regional levels
Identify and actively participate in media opportunities that call attention to the tobacco epidemic, including WNTD	Coordinate WNTD and other global/Regional media events that provide the opportunity to advocate for strong action against tobacco
Cooperate as appropriate to regularly collect and disseminate information on tobacco production, manufacture, sale and other activities of the tobacco industry which have an impact on the WHO FCTC or national tobacco control activities and regularly report to WHO	Establish and maintain a global system to regularly collect and disseminate information on tobacco production, manufacture, sale and other activities of the tobacco industry that may have an impact on the WHO FCTC or national tobacco control activities and regularly communicate results to Member States
Consistent with Article 20, institute research and public inquiries into tobacco industry activities and influence at country level	Provide technical and logistic support to Member States that request inquiries into tobacco industry activities

Conclusion

Controlling the tobacco epidemic in the Western Pacific requires strategic coordination, resources and political commitment. The WHO Framework Convention on Tobacco Control provides a global template for the minimum standards for best practice in tobacco control. Ensuring its ratification and entry into force is the first, and critical step, for Member States. Simultaneously, national capacity for tobacco control needs to be reinforced and developed further, to enable countries to implement the provisions of the Convention. The Convention provides the vision, but the Member States must supply the action, to reduce the harm caused by tobacco use and exposure to tobacco smoke.

Tobacco control is an ongoing process. This Regional Plan of Action takes the process a step further than the previous Action Plan. Whereas the 2000-2004 Plan outlined the basic elements for establishing national capacity to deal with the tobacco epidemic, this current plan directs Member States to consider the comprehensiveness of various interventions. Earlier Action Plans relied on external sources of support to fund country activities. However, this Plan encourages countries to seriously consider national mechanisms to ensure sustainability. Finally, this Plan promotes standardized regional mechanisms and instruments for surveillance, research, evaluation, information dissemination and advocacy.

Member States in the Western Pacific Region bear a disproportionate health and economic burden caused by tobacco use. Heightened advertising and promotion of tobacco products by the tobacco industry within the Region, and increased trade in tobacco products brought about by liberalization of trade agreements as Member States open up their markets to the forces of globalization connote an even higher toll in the future.

This Regional Plan of Action for Tobacco Control comes at an opportune moment, with the adoption of the international Framework Convention on Tobacco Control. The adoption of the Convention presents the Region with a crucial window of opportunity to make significant progress against the tobacco epidemic through the strategic alignment of national and regional efforts with the Convention.

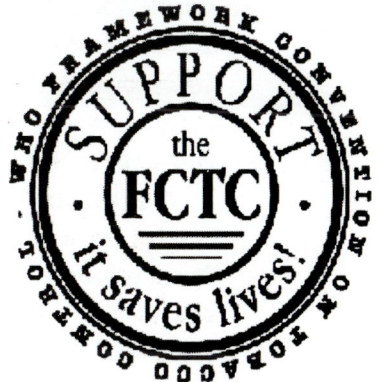

Continuation of conclusion

Member States have a chance to strengthen national programmes and interregional collaboration to effectively address what is fast becoming the single most preventable cause of early death and chronic disability. This opportunity should not be wasted. Too many lives in the Region have already been lost, and too many impoverished families are prevented from improving their lives, by tobacco.

Working together, the optimal approach to counter the tobacco epidemic in the Region can be established.

United, the Member States of the Western Pacific can achieve the vision of a tobacco free Region.

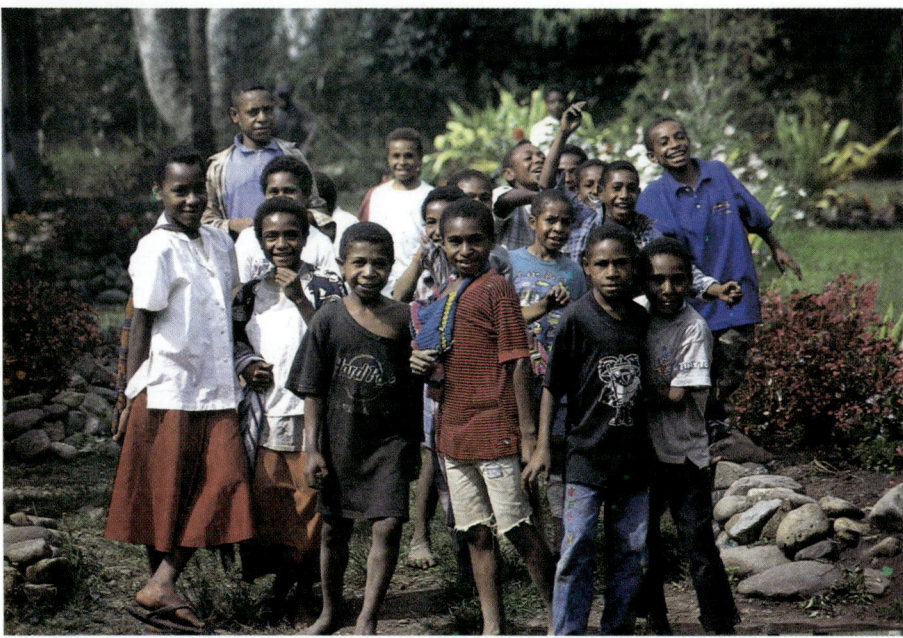

This Regional Action Plan is intended as a critical element to guide Member States towards the implementation of the provisions of the WHO Framework Convention on Tobacco Control. Through the strategic actions outlined in this plan, it is hoped that Member States will be able to join forces and effectively counter the tobacco epidemic.

Key references

Most of these references are available in full text on the Internet. If you need assistance in obtaining a hard copy of the reference, please contact your WHO country office or the Tobacco Free Initiative, WHO Western Pacific Regional Office (see contact information on the back cover).

General references

WHO Framework Convention on Tobacco Control
World Health Organization 2003
This WHO website contains information on the WHO Framework Convention on Tobacco Control, including the full text of the Convention and World Health Assembly resolution 56.1, with links to official translations in Arabic, Chinese, French, Russian, and Spanish.
http://www.who.int/entity/tobacco/framework

The Tobacco Atlas
World Health Organization 2002
WHO's tobacco atlas provides detailed data from countries on the differences and similarities of the global tobacco control struggle.
http://www.who.int/tobacco/resources/publications/tobacco_atlas/en/

Tobacco Control Country Profiles
Edited by Shafey O, Dolwick S, Guindon GE. Second Edition 2003
Collectively these country profiles present a composite picture of the status of the tobacco pandemic in the early 21st century.
http://www.who.int/tobacco/global_data/country_profiles/en/

Policy and economics research

Curbing the Epidemic: Governments and the Economics of Tobacco Control
World Bank 1999
This report outlines effective policy interventions to reduce smoking in developing countries. It discusses tobacco use and its consequences on both health and the economy, and highlights the relationship between smoking and poverty.
http://www1.worldbank.org/tobacco/reports.htm

Tobacco Control in Developing Countries
Curbing The Epidemic Governments And The Economics Of Tobacco Control draws on this book of background papers
Jha P and Chaloupka F. 2000
http://www1.worldbank.org/tobacco/tcdc.asp

Tobacco Control Policy: Strategies, Successes and Setbacks
Edited by Waverly Brigden L., de Beyer, J, World Bank 2003
This book contains the stories of six countries – Brazil, Bangladesh, Canada, Poland, South Africa, and Thailand. These countries, selected to provide global geographical representation, are in different stages of the tobacco epidemic and the strength and history of their tobacco control policies vary considerably. Each has achieved notable success in tobacco control policy-making, basing advocacy and policies on sound research and evidence.
http://publications.worldbank.org/ecommerce/catalog/product?item_id=1485821

Confronting the Tobacco Epidemic in an Era of Trade Liberalization
World Health Organization 2001
This paper examines the links between international trade liberalization and tobacco consumption. It explores new horizons for econometric and other economic research focusing on trade, investment and tobacco, and considers the legal and political issues involved in proposed efforts to address the liberalization of trade in tobacco within the WHO's Framework Convention on Tobacco Control.
http://whqlibdoc.who.int/hq/2001/WHO_NMH_TFI_01.4.pdf

Key references

Regulating tobacco products
The WHO Study Group on Tobacco Product Regulation (TobReg), formerly the Scientific Advisory Group on Tobacco, is a group of scientists in the fields of product regulation and laboratory analysis of tobacco ingredients and emissions, tasked with advising on effective and evidence-based means to achieve a coordinated regulatory framework for tobacco products. This website includes information and recommendations on regulating tobacco products, such a review of the role of toxicity testing in tobacco product testing, biomarkers of exposure and effect, and testing methods for smokeless tobacco.
http://www.who.int/tobacco/global_interaction/tobreg/en/

Epidemiological research

2004 United States Surgeon General's Report: The Health Consequences of Smoking
United States Department of Health and Human Services 2004
This website contains full text access to the *2004 Surgeon General's Report: The Health Consequences of Smoking*, as well as an interactive database that includes abstracts of more than 1600 key cited articles, and an interactive animation outlining the effects of smoking on the different organs of the body based on the findings of the 2004 Surgeon General's Report. The report reviews only active smoking.
http://www.cdc.gov/tobacco/sgr/sgr_2004/index.htm

IARC Monographs on the Evaluation of Carcinogenic Risks to Humans
The International Agency for Research on Cancer (IARC) is part of the World Health Organization. Its mission is to coordinate and conduct research on the causes of human cancer, the mechanisms of carcinogenesis, and to develop scientific strategies for cancer control.

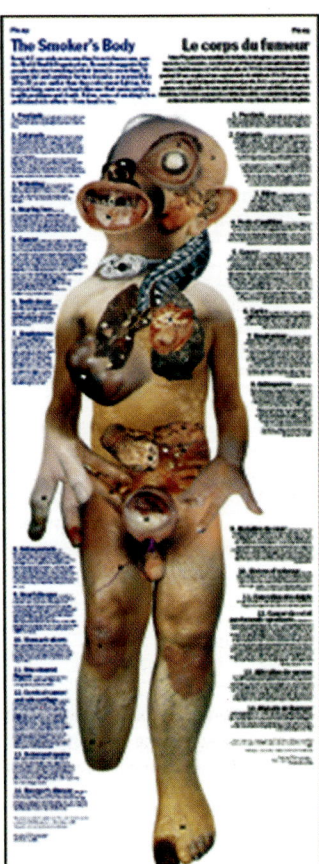

- **Tobacco Smoke and Involuntary Smoking**
  IARC Vol., 83, 2004
  IARC concludes that involuntary smoking (exposure to secondhand or 'environmental' tobacco smoke) is carcinogenic to humans.
  http://monographs.iarc.fr/htdocs/monographs/vol83/01-smoking.html
  http://www.iarc.fr/IARCPress/general/monographvol83.html

- **Betel-quid and Areca-nut Chewing**
  IARC, Vol. 85, 2004
  In many countries, particularly in the Asia Pacific region, unripe areca nut is chewed with slaked lime and betel inflorescence, sometimes wrapped in betel leaf. Tobacco is often added. In this monograph IARC concludes that betel quid with tobacco is *carcinogenic to humans, betel* quid without tobacco is *carcinogenic*
  to humans, and areca nut is carcinogenic to humans.
  http://www-cie.iarc.fr/htdocs/monographs/vol85/85-01-betel-areca.html

- **Smokeless Tobacco Products**
  IARC Vol. 89, 2004
  IARC concluded that smokeless tobacco is carcinogenic to humans.
  http://www.iarc.fr/ENG/Press_Releases/pr154a.html
  [Note: At the time of publication, this IARC monograph was in preparation. Access to the related published article, "Smokeless tobacco and tobacco-related nitrosamines" (Coglian V, et al. 2004) is available through free registration to The Lancet Oncology, Volume 5, Number 12, December 2004
  http://oncology.thelancet.com/journal

The Smoker's Body Poster
A poster showing some of the effects of tobacco use on health. Available online in English, French and Spanish.
http://www.who.int/tobacco/research/smokers_body/en/

Key references

Youth and women

Tobacco and the rights of the child
World Health Organization 2001
This paper examines the major problems posed by tobacco as they relate to the provisions of the Convention on the Rights of the Child, particularly in relation to civil rights and freedoms, basic health and welfare, and child labour.
http://www.who.int/tobacco/resources/publications/rights_child/en/

International Consultation on Environmental Tobacco Smoke (ETS) and Child Health
World Health Organization 2000
Experts from developed and developing countries examined the effects of ETS (secondhand smoke or passive smoking) on child health and recommended interventions to reduce these harmful effects and eliminate children's exposure.
http://www.who.int/entity/tobacco/research/en/ets_report.pdf

Women and the Tobacco Epidemic: Challenges for the 21st Century
World Health Organization 2001
This book supports a powerful and important concept - that the rights of women and children to health are basic human prerogatives.
http://whqlibdoc.who.int/hq/2001/WHO_NMH_TFI_01.1.pdf

Seeing Beneath the Surface: The Truth About the Tobacco Industry's Youth Smoking Prevention Programmes
World Health Organization 2002
A WHO brochure on the tobacco industry's efforts to promote ineffective youth smoking prevention programmes.
http://www.wpro.who.int/tfi/docs/PressReleases/Seeing_bneath_d_surface.pdf

Cessation

Policy Recommendations for Smoking Cessation and Treatment of Tobacco Dependence
Edited by da Costa e Silva, V. World Health Organization 2003
This publication was produced following the WHO meeting on Global Policy for Smoking Cessation, in Moscow, in June 2002, and includes recommendations that take into account countries' different national contexts, culture, health-care systems and financing capacity.
http://www.who.int/tobacco/resources/publications/tobacco_dependence/en/

Other

Towards Health With Justice
World Health Organization 2002
A review of litigation and public inquiries as tools for tobacco control.
http://www.who.int/entity/tobacco/media/en/final_jordan_report.pdf

Low Cost Research Advocacy
A guide for organizations and individuals to advocate for effective tobacco control.
Efroymson D. PATH Canada, August 2002
http://www.pathcanada.org/library/docs/Eng_res_Guide.pdf

Tobacco Industry Strategies to Undermine Tobacco Control Activities at the World Health Organization
World Health Organization 2001
Evidence from tobacco industry documents reveals that tobacco companies have operated for many years with the deliberate purpose of subverting the efforts of the World Health Organization to control tobacco use. The attempted subversion has been elaborate, well financed, sophisticated, and usually invisible.
http://www.who.int/tobacco/resources/publications/general/who_inquiry/en/

Key resources

These are only a small sampling of on-line resources for tobacco control information.

WHO's Tobacco Free Initiative
This website contains information on the Tobacco Free Initiative, established in July 1998 to focus international attention, resources and action on the global tobacco epidemic.
www.who.int/tobacco/en/

The World Bank Group: The Economics of Tobacco Control
This is an excellent World Bank website that contains:
- The full text of "Curbing the Epidemic: governments and the economics of tobacco control", 1999 World Bank report in English and other languages.
- All the background papers, published as "Tobacco Control in Developing Countries" 2000 (TCDC book).
- Short country profiles (notes and graphs) on tobacco production, trade, use, policies etc for many countries.
- PowerPoint presentations on tobacco and policies to reduce its harm (including talking notes). FAQs and common myths and facts about tobacco control.
- Tools that explain how to analyze tobacco demand, employment, smuggling, taxation, poverty issues.
- Effective interventions to reduce tobacco use at a glance.

www1.worldbank.org/tobacco/

GLOBALink, International Union Against Cancer's (UICC)
GLOBALink, UICC's tobacco control network, is a giant online communication tool for over 3500 tobacco control professionals. GLOBALink is a recognized catalyst for dialogue and collective action between tobacco control professionals.
www.globalink.org

Tobacco Control Online, *British Medical Journal*
On-line version of the *Tobacco Control Journal*, an international peer review journal for health professionals and others in tobacco control. Access to the full journal is by subscription, but free access is offered to developing countries.
tc.bmjjournals.com/

Tobacco Information and Prevention Source (TIPS), United States Centers for Disease Control and Prevention (CDC)
A comprehensive source of tobacco control information, including US Surgeon General Reports on tobacco related issues, research and surveillance and education materials.
www.cdc.gov/tobacco/index.htm

Clearinghouse for Tobacco Control, National Poison Centre of the Universiti Sains Malaysia
The Clearinghouse for Tobacco (C-Tob) was established to garner and disseminate information on tobacco control to all interested parties and readers focusing in particular on countries in South-East Asia.
www.prn2.usm.my/main.asp

VicHealth Centre for Tobacco Control
This site provides information about the centre and its research as well as links to important repositories of knowledge on tobacco control both ikn and outside Australia.
www.vctc.org.au/